Clinical Guide
for the Treatment of
Male Sexual Addiction

Syllabus for a Group Program with
Recovery From Sexual Addiction Books

Clinical Guide
for the Treatment of Male Sexual Addiction

Syllabus for a Group Program with Recovery From Sexual Addiction Books

Paul Becker, LPC

authorHOUSE®

AuthorHouse™
1663 Liberty Drive
Bloomington, IN 47403
www.authorhouse.com
Phone: 1-800-839-8640

Published by AuthorHouse 1/31/2013

ISBN: 978-1-4817-0996-5 (sc)
ISBN: 978-1-4817-1081-7 (e)

Any people depicted in stock imagery provided by Thinkstock are models, and such images are being used for illustrative purposes only.
Certain stock imagery © Thinkstock.

This book is printed on acid-free paper.

Because of the dynamic nature of the Internet, any web addresses or links contained in this book may have changed since publication and may no longer be valid. The views expressed in this work are solely those of the author and do not necessarily reflect the views of the publisher, and the publisher hereby disclaims any responsibility for them.

Table of Contents

This book: *Clinical Guide for the Treatment of Male Sexual Addiction* , is written for therapists/ counselors for use in a group clinical setting. It is an instructional guide on how to use the books:

Recovery From Sexual Addiction: A Man's Guide and

Recovery From Sexual Addiction: A Man's Workbook

These books help men to remove unwanted sexual behavior from their lives.

Both books may be purchased on-line from:

sexaddictionhelpbooks.com

Introduction

This guide is intended to facilitate the use of the book, *Recovery From Sexual Addiction: A Man's Guide* and the accompanying workbook in a sex addiction group program. It supports clinical therapists by providing interventions for men who wish to end addictive sexual behaviors. This intervention program can be summarized through the following statements: Vision, Program Goal and Objectives of Therapy.

Leading Vision: Assist men who are seeking answers in the right places.

Program Goal: Men who participate in this program will end lustful sexual thinking, fantasies and behavior.

Program Objective: Lead men through a structured clinical process intended to help them become aware and understand the complex factors that contribute to sexual addiction. The program objective is supported by exploring:

- The nature, characteristics, and factors underlying sexual addiction.

- The beginning of sexual addiction, often found in age-inappropriate exposure to sexual behavior or material.

- Age-inappropriate exposure to sexual behavior or material which causes feelings of sexual arousal, shame, and guilt. These confusing feelings together with a lack of fatherly emotional nourishment often form the roots of sexual addiction.

- Sexual addiction as a shame-based disease that began at a time of life when adult choices were not possible. The addict is not a bad person but is dealing with a bad problem.

- Sex addiction may take root in late teens or early adulthood after a significant first time, sexual exposure.

- Why a sexually-addicted man is not alone in his struggle. A substantial proportion of the male population struggles with elements of sexual addiction at some time during their lives.

- The challenges of overcoming compulsive addictive behavior as addressed through education and behavioral modification processes.

- How anger, anxiety, depressed mood, and isolation contribute to lustful thinking, fantasies, and behavior.

- How empowering men to exercise choice gives them hope of changing the sexual addiction dance.

- How recovery includes changing one's attachment to sexual fantasy, thinking, and behavior.

- How recovery includes changing one's life by coming out of isolation, taking steps to give up depressed mood, improving family relationships, and developing a support network.

- How recovery includes making and sustaining a high-level commitment to end lustful sexual thinking, fantasies, and behavior.

- Providing resources to support an addiction-free life journey.

Notes:

At least twenty to twenty-five weekly **90** minute sessions are needed to lead sexually-addicted men through the *Recovery from Sexual Addiction* books. This guide is not intended to be definitive in terms of the time needed to process each concept. The goal is not to complete the book and workbook. Working at a pace the group finds remedial is far more important. As such, it is within reason to add more sessions to your program. At times the counselor will find it prudent to attend to one or more unplanned agendas brought to the session by group members. Little or no progress is made in the text or workbook during some sessions. Also, adding supplemental material to the program is often helpful to the progress of the group.

All group members should be encouraged to attend a Twelve-Step Program. Appendix A of the book, *Recovery from Sexual Addiction: A Man's Guide*, lists Twelve-Step Programs for sexually-addicted men.

Completing the book and workbook will not assure universal cessation of sexually acting-out behavior. Each man progresses on his own internal timetable. For some, ending acting-out behavior comes quickly but for others, progress is slower. It is not usual for men to repeat the program. Addiction experts Patrick Carnes and John Bradshaw believe the healing process spans years. At the conclusion of the program all group members are encouraged to continue their healing journey through individual and marital counseling as well as continued attendance at Twelve-Step Program(s).

Clinical Considerations for Mental Health Professionals

- This program has been developed for men. There is no clinical experience to suggest that this particular program is effective for women.

- Before a man attends his first group session, schedule one or more individual therapy sessions to determine his suitability for the group process, that is, will he contribute to and benefit by the program. During an individual session(s) encourage the man to disclose the full scope of his sexual history and current acting-out behavior. During the group program, while men are encouraged to disclose the nature of their acting-out behavior, they are not encouraged to provide details that may be toxic to another man in the group. In some cases, full disclosure during the group process may become a source of new behavior for another member of the group. Certain aberrant behaviors such as sex with animals or children go beyond reasonable norms of group disclosure. Certain sexual behaviors are best processed during one-on-one therapy. Keep in mind you may be legally obligated to report sexual behavior that involves children.

- Consistent weekly on-time attendance is an important task for group members. Establish a policy that members pay for unexcused absences.

- It is not unusual for one or more of the group members to have a public persona. Group members need to guarantee confidentiality to their fellow travelers.

- Ideally it is desirable to begin the program with a sufficient number of participants so that the group can be closed to new members. Notwithstanding this ideal, a man who enters the program after it has begun can still gain insights to help him change his sexual behavior. If a man enters the group halfway through the program, encourage him to stay with the program when the next series of sessions begin.

- Consider dedicating the first part of the session to "check-in." During check-in each man is invited to share his status on his recovery journey.

- Early in the program the dialog is between group members and the clinical counselor. After cohesion is formed in the group, constructive crosstalk should be encouraged.

- Ask group members to read assigned materials and complete written assignments between sessions. Use the session to discuss important concepts. Unfortunately, the "ideal" doesn't always happen. You may find that reading the text aloud during sessions is needed to keep group members on the same page. After every few paragraphs or at the end of a subsection, ask members a question about the material just read. For example, "Did you identify with…?" or "Share your feelings about…" Sometimes the discussion is short, but at other times the group strikes a golden understanding. Go with the gold!

- Despite encouragement and promises, written assignments are not always completed between sessions. Some men prefer to come early each week to complete written assignments. A less preferable option is to allot time to complete written exercises during the group session.

- The workbook requires men to record information they may find embarrassing and shameful. Some fear family members or others may read the answers they provide. You may decide to have workbook exercises completed just prior to the session or during a session and to collect the workbooks at the end of each session and give them back at the following session. If you retain members' workbooks between sessions, confidentiality should be pledged. It is more important for each man to get in touch with the full range of his past and addictive practices than updating the counselor's knowledge, at least early on in the program. It takes time to lift the veil of shame.

- The majority of men enter therapy because their sexual behavior has been "found out" by their spouses. It is common and understandable for a spouse to react harshly to learning that her partner has not respected the marriage contract. In these situations encourage the spouse to schedule an individual therapy session. During the session empower the spouse to ask questions about sexual addiction. A spouse may find reading the book, *Why Is My Partner Sexually Addicted: Insight Women Need* by Paul Becker, enlightening.

- Men and women see the world differently. Sexually-addicted men are driven to repeat the good feelings associated with "orgasm," whereas women see sex as part of a "relationship" commitment. A woman, rightfully, cannot understand how her partner can "do his thing," and be committed to the marriage. While women have the correct concept, it will take the male time to alter his thinking. Ask her to give her man time to heal. In time, hopefully, he will see the world as she does.

- Frequently, sexually-addicted men have codependent marriages. Suggest to spouses that her partner needs an accountability partner to whom he is not married. Each partner needs time to work on his or her own issues. Freeing the spouse of the burden of accountability is preferred.

- Men often feel that once they have pleaded sorrow for their behavior, trust should be restored to the marriage. The couple needs to understand that ending unwanted sexual behavior is rarely an instant decision and trust is only gained through prolonged sobriety and a changed lifestyle. Encourage spouses to read *Why Is My Partner Sexually Addicted: Insight Women Need,* by Paul Becker, *Don't Call It Love,* by Patrick Carnes, and *Getting the Love You Want,* by Harville Hendrix.

Note: For the sexually-addicted man, much of the information in *Recovery From Sexual Addiction: A Man's Guide* and its accompanying workbook is new to him. Certain important concepts are treated more than once. It takes more than one pass to internalize and apply important new concepts.

A syllabus for a twenty-week group therapy program follows. It is intended to be a fluid guide that can be revised and extended to suit the needs to the group.

GROUP PROGRAM
Session One

Goal: Introduction of the program	Material needed: Handout - 2 Corinthians 12:7-10
Objective: Establish group norms and begin to expose shame.	Introduction to Group Program

Brief discussion of consent and disclosure form: Ask each person to sign your form.

Brief discussion of the group norms and process:

- Discuss attendance, participation, on-time presence, expressing feelings, respectful confrontation, honesty, use of "I" statements ("I feel disrespected when people start whispering while I'm talking."), disclosure, dominating discussion vs. holding back, intellectualizing, confidentiality (what is said in the room stays in the room), disclosure of sensitive information about self, roles of a group leader (teacher, counselor/therapist, and supporter), and cost of the group sessions.

- The group program is a combination of education and therapy. It is not a Twelve-Step program. All group members are encouraged to attend a relevant sex addiction Twelve-Step program. See Appendix A in the book for a listing.

- The program structure facilitates understanding self, the nature of sexual addiction, and how one's life can be changed to reduce the influence of addiction.

- Therapeutic expectations: Ask group members to be patient and trust in the process. Unwanted sexual behavior did not begin overnight and recovery will take time. For some, it may take the rest of their lives. We don't talk in terms of a cure, but in terms of a recovery journey.

- Recovery takes commitment and much work. In order to cover much ground, homework is assigned. It is essential, as a first commitment, for group members to complete their between session assignments with considerable thought.

- Addictions come in various shapes and sizes. What is important is how the addiction affects an individual's life. Ask group members not to compare themselves to others. No one has an accurate measuring stick. If another man's sexual behavior seems more severe, ask them to have empathy for him.

Introductions: Pair each man with another. Ask members to exchange information in order to report to the whole group about their partner. Ask the men to report on the following information: name, something important about the person, and a personal goal the partner has for group counseling. Record goals on large sheets of paper or on a white board.

Draw feelings: Ask each man to take a piece of paper and draw on one half a symbol or picture of how he feels as he comes into the group. On the other half, draw a symbol or picture how he hopes to feel after he ends his acting-out behaviors. Ask group members to share their thinking and feelings.

Discussion of humanness: We are not alone in our failings—several of the apostles had great difficulties. Ask the men to discuss their understanding of 2 Corinthians **12:7-10**:

> *To keep me from becoming conceited because of these surpassingly great revelations, there was given me a thorn in my flesh, a messenger of Satan, to torment me. Three times I pleaded with the Lord to take it away from me. But he said to me, "My grace is sufficient for you, for my power is made perfect in weakness." Therefore I will boast all the more gladly about my weaknesses, so that Christ's power may rest on me. That is why, for Christ's sake, I delight in weaknesses, in insults, in hardships, in persecutions, in difficulties. For when I am weak, then I am strong.*

The Apostle Paul, who wrote the above words, had a "thorn" in his side. What the thorn represented is unknown but we do know it troubled him -- could it have been an addiction?

Between-session assignment: Ask each man to recall two choices he currently faces. Suggest one choice be related to sexual behavior and note the factors affecting his choices. Ask group members to be prepared to discuss their answers at the next session.

Handouts: 2 Corinthians **12:7-10**.

Homework assignment: Read Chapter One of the book, *Recovery From Sexual Addiction: A Man's Guide*

End with the Serenity Prayer See page **80** of the book.

GROUP PROGRAM
Sessions Two and Three

Goal: Educate	Material needed: Book, *Recovery From Sexual Addiction: A Man's Guide*
Objective: Provide an understanding of sexual addiction and its characteristics.	Chapter: One

Report on between-session assignment: Ask each man to report on two choices he is facing and what are his alternatives. Include one choice related to sexual behavior. What are the factors affecting his choices?

From Chapter One of the book:

Page #	Action: Read and discuss.	
1-3 Book	Primary Topic: What Is Sexual Addiction?	The purpose of this section is to introduce the concept of sexual addiction.
	Discussion Topic:	Discussion Points:
1-3 Book	What is sexual addiction? Ben's Story	Ask group members: • To share their feelings when they hear the term "sexual addiction." • If they identify with any of the material presented.

From Chapter One of the book:

Page #	Action: Read and discuss.	
3-8 Book	Primary Topic: Common Characteristics of Unwanted Sexual Behavior.	The purpose of this section is to introduce some common characteristics of unwanted sexual behavior.
	Discussion Topics:	Discussion Points:
3 Book	Multiple practices.	No discussion is needed.

Paul Becker, LPC

3-4 Book	Obsession	Ask group members to discuss, "Sex has become my greatest need." Ask for examples.
4-5 Book	Practices become compulsive and unmanageable.	Ask group members to share how their sexual behavior has become unmanageable.
6 Book	Tolerance	Ask group members to discuss: " I keep looking for a new high and don't find it."
7 Book	Progression	Ask the men to discuss: "I am curious and I look to engage in new and exciting sexual activities."
7 Book	Withdrawal	Ask group members to discuss: • "I fear giving up my best friend (sex)." • "My brain tells me, 'I want more.'"
7 Book	Life-damaging consequences.	Ask group members to share the negative consequences of sexual addiction in their lives.
8 Book	Change in life focus.	Ask group members to share how sexual addiction has become a primary motivator, a primary need.
8 Book	Sex addiction cycle and rituals.	No discussion is needed. Just recognize that sex addiction cycles and rituals exist and will be addressed later.
8 Book	Denial.	Ask group members for examples of illogical thinking they use to justify sexual behavior.

From Chapter One of the book:

Page #	**Action:** Read	
8-10 Book	**Primary Topic:** Unwanted Sexual Behaviors Found in the *Diagnostic and Statistical Manual of Mental Disorders, Fourth Edition (DSM-IV-TR)*.	The purpose of this section is to introduce sexual addiction behaviors that are considered "paraphilias" by the mental health profession.
	Discussion Topic:	**Discussion Points:**
8-10 Book	Unwanted sexual behaviors.	Ask group members to read this section to themselves. It is enough for group members to understand that paraphilias exist and some members may identify with one or more. However, a discussion of paraphilias at this stage of the program should be done in individual therapy, if needed.

| 4 |

From Chapter One of the book:

Page #	**Action:** Read and discuss.	
10 Book	**Primary Topic:** Unwanted Sexual Behaviors Not Found in the *DSM-IV-TR*.	The purpose of this section is to introduce the sexual addiction behaviors that are often addressed in therapy but are not considered "paraphilias."
	Discussion Topic:	**Discussion Points:**
10 Book	More unwanted sexual behaviors	Ask group members to read this section to themselves. Ask if there are questions. Discuss as needed.

From Chapter One of the book:

Page #	**Action:** Read and discuss.	
10-11 Book	**Primary Topic:** Compulsive Sexual Behaviors.	The purpose of this section is to introduce the compulsive sexual behaviors which are frequently addressed in therapy.
	Discussion Topics:	**Discussion Points:**
11 Book	Masturbation. Pornography. Cybersex. Phone Sex.	Ask group members if they identify with any of the enumerated behaviors. Discussion should be brief but enough to foster awareness.

From Chapter One of the book:

Page #	**Action:** Read and discuss.	
11-17 Book	**Primary Topic:** Underlying Factors of Sexual Addiction.	The purpose of this section is to introduce underlying factors that often lead to or support sexual addiction.
	Discussion Topics:	**Discussion Points:**
11-12 Book	Were you sexually abused as a child or adolescent?	Ask group members how they identify with the following factors. Discussion should be brief but enough to foster awareness.

12 Book	Do you regularly purchase sexually explicit magazines?	
12 Book	Do you regularly pursue online pornography?	
13 Book	Are you often preoccupied with sexual thoughts?	
13 Book	What is the problem? Don't all people have sexual memories?	
13 Book	Does your spouse or significant other ever worry or complain about your sexual behavior?	
13-14 Book	Can you stop your sexual behavior when you know it's inappropriate?	
14 Book	Do you ever feel badly about your sexual behavior?	
14 Book	Has sexual behavior ever created problems for you or your family?	
14-15 Book	Do you worry about people finding out about this behavior?	
15 Book	Do you lead a double life?	
15 Book	Do you keep secrets about your sexual or romantic activities from those important to you?	
15 Book	Has your behavior ever emotionally hurt someone?	
16 Book	Are any of your sexual activities against the law (for example, sex with minors or exposure of genitals in public)?	
16 Book	Have you ever felt degraded by your sexual activity?	
16 Book	Do you feel depressed after having sex?	

16 Book	Do you fear sexual intimacy? Do you avoid sex at all costs?	
16-17 Book	Do you frequently feel remorse, shame, or guilt after a sexual encounter?	
17 Book	Have you ever tried to limit or stop masturbating?	
17 Book	Do you lose your sense of identity or meaning in life without sex or a love relationship?	
17 Book	Does your pursuit of sex or romantic relationships interfere with your spiritual development?	

From Chapter One of the book:

Page #	**Action:** Read and discuss.	
17-19 Book	**Primary Topic:** Insights into Sexual Addiction.	The purpose of this section is to introduce another author's insights into sexual addiction.
	Discussion Topic:	**Discussion Points:**
17-19 Book	Insights into sexual addiction.	Ask group members: • What statements are of interest. • Do they identify with any of the statements. • If they have questions.

Discuss key points group members learned from this chapter. Insights gained become the fuel for changed behavior.

Handouts: None.

Homework assignment: Read and complete exercises from Chapter One of the workbook.

End with the Serenity Prayer. See page **80** of the book.

GROUP PROGRAM
Session Four

Goal: Penetrate shame and denial.	Material needed: Guide and Workbook, *Recovery From Sexual Addiction* books
Objective: Gain deeper understanding of one's addiction.	Chapter: One

From Chapter One of the workbook:

Page #	Action: Read and discuss.	
1-3 Workbook	**Primary Topic:** Men's Stories.	The purpose of this section is to introduce other men's stories to help group members understand they did not invent the sexual addiction wheel.
	Discussion Topics:	**Discussion Points:**
1-3 Workbook	Andre's Story. Neil's Story. David's Story. Mike's Story. Ted's Story. Tony's Story. George's Story. James' Story.	Ask group members: • If they identify with any of the stories presented. • To share their feelings when they identify with another man's story. (Are they relieved to find others have had the same problem?)

From Chapter One of the workbook:

Page #	Action: Read, do the exercises, and discuss.	
3 Workbook	**Primary Topic:** How about You?	The purpose of this exercise is for each man to get in touch with the magnitude and impact of his sexual behaviors.

	Discussion Topics:	**Discussion Points:**
4-20 Workbook	Pornography. Masturbation. Sexual fantasy and thinking. Sexual encounters. Other sexual activities.	Ask group members: • To complete their sexual inventory. • To share their answers as they feel comfortable in doing so. • If they discovered anything new when they completed their inventory. • To share shame or guilt feelings they experienced while completing their inventory. **Note:** Some group members find completing a sex behavior inventory helpful and revealing. However, for some it is an embarrassing task. As such, it may take time for each man to fully disclose his sexual history. Gaining awareness, facing reality, and exposing denial are important tasks for group members. As disclosure progresses, shame will begin to diminish.
20 Workbook	Legality.	Talk about the risks of using a work based computer to view sexual media.
21-24 Workbook	Your story.	**Note:** This section is for men whose sexual behavior does not fit a listed category, for example, one of the paraphilias or bestiality.

From Chapter One of the workbook:

Page #	**Action:** Read, do the exercises, and discuss.	
25-27 Workbook	**Primary Topic:** Sexual Addiction Questions.	The purpose of this section is to explore sexual addiction corollaries as they relate to each man.
	Discussion Topics:	**Discussion Points:**
25 Workbook	Have your sexual practices become compulsive and unmanageable?	Ask group members to share past efforts to end acting-out behavior and the results.

25 Workbook	Have you experienced life-damaging consequences as a result of your sexual behavior?	Ask group members: • Is isolation a primary consequence? • To discuss other consequences including self-loathing, depression, anxiety, anger, despair, pervasive feelings of hopelessness, moral uncertainty, and broken relationships with family and God.
25 Workbook	Has your sexual addiction caused a change in your life focus?	Ask group members if sexual behavior has become a primary motivator, a primary need.
26 Workbook	Is keeping your sexual behavior a secret very important to you?	Ask group members how secrecy keeps the addicted man bound to addiction.
26 Workbook	Do you fear giving up your sexual behavior?	Ask group members if they fear giving up cherished sexual behavior, an old and familiar friend. **Note:** This is an important insight for group members.
26 Workbook	Have you denied that you have a sexual addiction problem?	At this stage several group members may be questioning if they are sexually addicted. Ask group members to share their thinking.
26-27 Workbook	What lies and excuses do you use to continue your sexual behavior?	Ask group members to: • Complete the exercises. • Share "lies and excuses" they use to justify sexual behavior. **Note:** Post answers to newsprint or a board. It is important for group members to realize that "lies and excuses" facilitate addiction.

From Chapter One of the workbook:

Page #	**Action:** Read, do the exercises, and discuss.	
28-30 Workbook	**Primary Topic:** Am I Sexually Addicted?	The purpose of this section is to penetrate denial.

	Discussion Topics:	Discussion Points:
28 Workbook	Am I sexually addicted? questions.	Ask group members to: • Complete the exercises. • Share answers to the question(s) • Yes, No, Maybe I am sexually addicted. Why?
29-30 Workbook	I have examined my unwanted sexual behaviors and determined that I want to change…	Ask group members to: • Complete the exercises. • Share their answers. **Note:** Answers may be unrealistic at this point. The purpose is to help group members begin to think about change.

Discuss key points group members learned from this chapter (End of workbook Chapter One). Insights gained become the fuel for changed behavior.

Handouts: None.

Homework Assignment: Read and complete Chapter Two from the book and Chapter Three in the workbook.

End with the Serenity Prayer. See page **80** of the book.

Goal: Penetrating shame by understanding sexual addiction was initially not a choice.	Material needed: book and workbook, *Recovery From Sexual Addiction* books
Objective: Gain deeper understanding of one's sexual addiction roots which began in childhood.	Chapters: Two (book) Three (workbook)

From Chapter Two of the book and Three from the workbook:

Page #	Action: Read, do the exercises, and discuss.	
22-27 Book	Primary Topic: Sexual Addiction Often Begins in Childhood.	The purpose of this section is to introduce the conditions that often form the root of sexual addiction in a story form.
	Discussion Topics:	Discussion Points:
22-27 Book	Jack's Story. Ted's Story. Hank's Story. Art's Story. Simon's Story. Jimmy's Story	Ask group members to read and consider the conditions that fostered sexual addiction in the men in each vignette.
38-40 Workbook		Note: If needed, supplement by reading "Mark's Story" and related questions on pages **38-40** of the workbook.
27-29 Book	Common elements in the above vignettes.	Ask group members to: • Complete the exercises. • Identify the conditions that fostered sexual addiction from the vignettes. • Discuss the conditions.

| 41-44 Workbook | Common elements in your life. Your Story | Ask group members:
 • Complete the exercises.
 • Identify the conditions that formed each group member's sexual addiction.
 • Allow each group member to present his story (not all can).
 • To identify their "*catalytic event.*" (Age-inappropriate exposure is referred to as a *catalytic event* or a *catalytic story.*)

 Note: It is common for some group members to have difficulty recalling their story. Hearing other men recall their stories may trigger memories. For some, memories will be unsettling. Memories of experiencing or causing abuse may require individual counseling. |

From Chapter Two of the workbook:

Page #	**Action:** Read, do the exercises, and discuss.	
20 Book and **45** Workbook	**Primary Topic:** Sexual Addiction Can Begin in Teenage or Early Adulthood.	The purpose of this section is to introduce the conditions that form the root of sexual addiction when the addiction begins in teen years or early adulthood.
	Discussion Topics:	**Discussion Points:**
20 Book	Sexual addiction can begin after childhood.	Ask group members if they identify with this scenario.
20-21 Book and **45** Workbook	Elijah's Story Abbot's Story Joshua's Story - an alternative story.	Ask group members to: • Identify the conditions that fostered sexual addiction in each vignette. • Discuss how conditions experienced by these men differ from those experienced by children who are exposed to age-inappropriate sexual material/ behavior during childhood.

46 Workbook	Your Story - an alternative story.	Ask group members to: • Complete the exercises. • Identify the conditions that fostered sexual addiction. • Discuss the events. **Note:** If all group members report that they experienced childhood exposure to age-inappropriate sexual material/ behavior, skip this section.

From Chapter Two of the book:

Page #	**Action:** Read and discuss.	
31-37 Book	**Primary Topic:** Highlight the Origin of Sexual Addiction.	The purpose of this section is to foster more discussion of the origin of sexual addiction and to firmly set in the minds of group members that they did not ask to be sexually addicted. **Note:** Long-term recovery is aided by a diminution of the shame associated with sexual addiction. Men cannot change what has happened to them, but they can choose, as adults, to stop experiencing pain rooted in childhood.
	Discussion Topics:	**Discussion Points:**
32 Book	Age-inappropriate exposure to sexual behavior or material.	Ask group members: • What was the consequence of their age-inappropriate exposure? • To discuss sexual behavior they adopted subsequently to exposure. • How did such behavior progress during teen and adult life. • To discuss their feelings when they experienced abuse.

32-34 Book	Family environment and structure.	Ask group members to: • Share whether their family environment met their childhood need for affection and emotional nourishment. If not, why not? • Assess their family as rigid or chaotic. • Share how their family environment contributed to living in isolation? • Share if they feel isolated today. • Discuss feelings generated by isolation. • Discuss how their family environment fed their addiction. • Share feelings associated with growing up in their family. **Note:** Not all men who are exposed to unwanted sexual material or acts become sexual addicted. The relationship between the child and parent makes a significant difference.
34-35 Book	Arousal.	Ask group members to: • Share how well they remember their catalytic event. Ask why they can't remember what was served on one's birthday that year—another special occasion. • Discuss why the *catalytic event* was encoded in their brain. (It was one of the defining moments of life.) • Discuss feelings associated with arousal… excitement, shame, guilt, confusion, etc.
35-36 Book	Feelings of shame, guilt, and depression.	Ask group members to: • Discuss the difference between feeling guilty and ashamed. • Relate why their addiction fostered feelings of shame, guilt, and depressed mood. • Discuss why loving marital relations are not accompanied by similar feelings. • Discuss why shame fuels sexual compulsivity (need to medicate depressed mood and other negative feelings). • Discuss if depressed mood plays a role in their lives.

36 Book	Learned model in childhood repeated in adulthood.	Ask group members if they repeat behaviors first began in childhood. Why?
36-37 Book	Richard's Story.	Ask group members if: • They identify with the conditional love experienced by Richard. • Sexual behaviors were passed down from one generation to the next in their family. • They will pass their sexual addiction on to their children. Ask group members: • To share memories of conditional love from their families of origin. • To describe how it felt to be loved conditionally. • In what way do group members love their children conditionally.

Discuss key points group members learned from this chapter (end of the workbook Chapter Three) Insights gained become the fuel for changed behavior.

Handouts: None.

Homework Assignment: Read and complete Chapters Three from the book and Four from the workbook.

End with the Serenity Prayer. See page **80** of the book.

GROUP PROGRAM
Sessions Seven, Eight, and Nine

Goal: Understanding the sobriety challenge.	**Material needed:** book and workbook, *Recovery From Sexual Addiction* books
Objective: Gain deeper understanding of the complexity of sexual addiction.	**Chapter:** Three (book) Four (workbook)

From Chapter Three of the book and Chapter Four of the workbook:

Page #	**Action:** Read, do the exercises and discuss.	
38-40 Book	**Primary Topic:** Brain Indoctrination.	The purpose of this section is to explain how sexual addiction has changed the brain.
	Discussion Topic:	**Discussion Points:**
38-39 Book	Habit.	Ask group members: • If they habitually repeat their sexual thinking, fantasy, and behavior. • To discuss how sex becomes the addict's number one focus—his number one need.
49-51 Workbook		**Note:** Supplement with the exercises under, "Altering the Brain and Forming a Habit," on pages **49-51** of the workbook.

39 Book	Sexual fantasies.	Ask group members: • To discuss how sexual thinking and fantasy precede acting out. • If they agree that their sexual fantasies are part of their brain's indoctrination and serve as a launching platform for acting out. • Why not just stop sexual thinking and fantasy if it is the precursor to acting out? Discuss why it is difficult to stop. **Note:** Supplement with "Sexual Fantasies" exercises on pages **52-54** of the workbook. Ultimately, a commitment to change involves gaining control over the mind. Ask group members: • To examine how sexual fantasies play a key role in continuing acting-out behaviors. • Share their exercise answers.
52-54 Workbook		
39-40 Book	Altering the brain.	Ask group members: • If their brain now considers repetitive sexual stimulation normal. • Why does the brain encourage repetition of sexual activity to generate pleasurable feelings. • To discuss why the brain remembers euphoria related to orgasm.
40 Book	Association of systems.	Ask group members to share and name the associations that precede their acting-out behavior.
55-56 Workbook	Your sexually acting-out environment.	Ask group members: • How their environment supports their acting-out behavior. • To name their environmental triggers.
55 Workbook	Jude's Story.	Ask group members in what way do they identify with Jude's Story.
55-56 Workbook	Your Story.	Ask group members to complete the exercise and share how their environment supports acting-out behavior.

From Chapter Three of the book:

Page #	Action: Read and discuss.	
40-42 Book	**Primary Topic:** Isolation.	The purpose of this section is to explain how isolation is toxic to the sexually- addicted man.
	Discussion Topics:	**Discussion Points:**
40-41 Book	Hiding behind the mask.	Ask group members: • What does it mean to hide behind a mask for the sexually-addicted man? • What would taking off the mask look like? • How does one become vulnerable, that is, come out of isolation by sharing the "real person behind the mask?"
41 Book	Loneliness to isolation.	Ask group members: • Is the price of isolation loneliness? • How does childhood isolation spill over into adulthood? • If they feel lonely in their marriage. • How can feelings of loneliness be changed?
41 Book	Codependency.	Defer discussion of codependency until Session Ten where codependency is fully addressed.
42 Book	Sex to medicate pain.	Ask group members: • If they use sex to deal with life's problems and pain. • What life conditions are medicated? • Is medicating pain through sex linked to isolation?
42 Book	Sexual abuse as a child.	Ask group members: • To briefly discuss any new insights into how the combination of age-inappropriate sexual stimulus and dysfunctional family life is a formula for isolation and addiction. • If it is time to give up the childhood thinking and behavior and make an adult decision to change. • What would it look like to come out of isolation?

From Chapter Four of the workbook:

Page #	Action: Read, do the exercises and discuss.	
57-61 Workbook	**Primary Topic:** Acting-out Ritual.	The purpose of this section is to explain how sexual addiction is based on predictable ritual patterns.
	Discussion Topics:	**Discussion Points:**
57-58 Workbook	Tom's acting-out ritual.	Ask group members to: • Read Tom's acting-out ritual. • Identify points where Tom could have ended his ritual. • How does Tom deceive himself?
59-61 Workbook	Your acting-out rituals.	Ask group members to: • Complete the exercises (most men have multiple rituals). • Share their acting-out rituals. • Examine early points in the ritual(s) where an intervention could be successful. • Express their feelings at each step of their ritual.
45-46 Book	Greg's Story	**Note:** Supplement by reading, "Greg's Story." Establish an understanding that most sexual behavior is accompanied by a ritual. Ultimately the goal is to recognize the early steps of the ritual and to reject them.

From Chapter Four of the workbook:

Page #	Action: Read, do the exercises and discuss.	
62-66 Workbook	**Primary Topic:** Sex Addiction Cycle.	The purpose of this section is to explain the sexual addict's acting-out cycle.

	Discussion Topics:	Discussion Points:
62 Workbook	Sex Addiction Cycle	Ask group members to read the introduction to Sex Addiction Cycle.
63 Workbook	Initial phase—life condition.	Ask group members to: Read the initial phase—life condition. • Record and discuss one's own life conditions and the reason why this is the beginning of the acting-out cycle. • What changes in feelings or mood do they identify at the beginning of phase one? • Identify early feelings or changes in mood that could be addressed to preclude the acting-out cycle.
64 Workbook	Phase two—reaction to life condition.	Ask group members to: • Read phase two—reaction to life condition. • Record and discuss one's reaction to one's own life conditions. • Identify the reason this reaction contributes to the repetition of the acting-out cycle.
65 Workbook	Phase three—acting-out.	Ask group members to: • Read phase three—acting out. • Record and disclose an example of one's own acting-out ritual.

66 Workbook	Phase four—reconciliation	Ask group members to: Read phase four—reconciliation. <ul><li>Record and discuss one's own feelings of shame and guilt.</li><li>Record thinking that allows one to reject feelings of shame and guilt in order not to repeat the cycle.</li></ul> **Note:** Establish an understanding that sexually-addicted men repeat their acting-out cycles. Ultimately the goal is to recognize early steps within the cycle and choose alternative thinking and environments to reject repeating the acting-out cycle. Men seeking recovery often put more time between their addiction cycles. Increasing time between acting-out behaviors only constitutes longer cycles, not recovery.

Discuss key points group members learned from this chapter (end of the workbook Chapter Four). Insights gained become the fuel for changed behavior.

Handouts: None.

Homework Assignment: Read and complete Chapters Four and Five of the book and Chapter Six of the workbook.

End with the Serenity Prayer. See page **80** of the book.

Goal: Evaluating a broader aspect of the sexual addiction picture.	Material needed: book and workbook, *Recovery From Sexual Addiction* books
Objective: Gain a deeper understanding of how pornography and co-dependency impact sexual addiction.	Chapter: Four and Five (book) Six (workbook)

From Chapter Four of the book:

Page #	Action: Read and discuss.	
48-54 Book	**Primary Topic:** Pornography.	The purpose of this section is to understand that viewing pornography is the most common behavior of sexually-addicted men.
	Discussion Topics:	**Discussion Points:**
48-49 Book	Bart's Story. Bill's Story. Art's Story.	Ask group members: • If they identify with any of the behaviors found in these stories. • To share their behaviors related to viewing pornography.
50-51 Book	Definition of pornography.	Ask group members to enumerate the types of pornographic media they have used.
51-52 Book	Statistics on pornography.	Ask group members to: • Discuss statistics they find more shocking. • Share which statistics appear to be extreme. • Share which statistics seem to understate reality. • Share at what age they began to view pornography. • Share how frequently they access on-line pornography. • Share if they viewed pornography on a work computer.
53 Book	Internet pornography content.	Ask group members to share the nature and content of pornography that they view on line.

From Chapter Five of the book and Chapter Six of the workbook:

Page #	Action: Read, do the exercises and discuss.	
55 Book	**Primary Topic:** Codependency in marriage.	The purpose of this section is to introduce codependency factors that need to be addressed as part of recovery from sexual addiction.
	Discussion Topics:	**Discussion Points:**
55-56 Book	Codependency background.	Ask group members to read the background on page **55** of the book.
56 Book	Codependency in marriages where the male is sexually addicted.	Ask group members: • Why do sexually-addicted men tend to marry into a codependent relationship? • Why are both husband and wife likely to exhibit codependency characteristics? • Do men and women marry at the same level of childhood induced dysfunction?
57 Book	Who is to blame.	Ask group members why the "blame game" is counterproductive.
57-58 Book	Codependency characteristics are often evident before marriage. Jim and Barbara's Story	How do group members relate to Jim? Is he a realistic person? If so, why?
58-59 Book	Codependency characteristics flourish in marriage.	How do group members relate to Jim and Barbara's situation? Are they a realistic couple? If so, why?
59 **Book**	Epilog	Ask group members why Jim and Barbara's expectations of one another were doomed.
60 Book	Codependency characteristics in Jim and Barbara's marriage. Origin of codependency is found in a child's dysfunctional family.	Ask group members if they believe that men who are sexually-addicted and their spouses tend to come from dysfunctional families. If so, why?
61 Book	Children of codependent dysfunctional families have ill-formed or incomplete personalities.	Ask group members if they agree that codependency is passed from one generation to the next.

61 Book	In marriage, codependency fosters pain and negativity.	Ask group members if they find the same pain and negativity described in Jim and Barbara's marriage in their own marriages.
62 Book	Fear, shame, anger, and depressed mood are all companions of codependency.	Ask group members if they find fear, shame, anger, and depressed mood in their own marriages.
62 Book	Codependency is part of the problem.	Ask group members if they believe that Jim and Barbara's marriage can be saved.
62-63 Book	Joe and Alice's Story.	Ask group members: How they relate to Joe and Alice. What characteristics from Joe and Alice's Story tend to repeat in their marriages?
63 Book	The other side of the coin.	Do group members feel that the steps Alice took to reclaim her partner would be effective. Why?
64 Book	The answer.	If each group member was an "Alice," what would Alice's reaction be to the answer.
64 Book	A visual picture of Joe and Alice's codependency relationship.	Ask group members if they identify with the "elevator" analogy. If so, how?
64-65 Book	What needs to change?	Ask group members how they would change the "elevator" analogy in their marriages
65 Book	You and codependency addressed.	Ask group members if they want to read more on codependency.
96-99 Workbook	Codependency exercises	Ask group members to: Complete the exercise. Discuss insights gained.

Discuss key points group members learned from Chapters Four and Five in the book and Chapter Six in the workbook.

Handouts: None.

Homework Assignment: Read and complete Chapters Six from the book and Chapter Five in the workbook.

End with the Serenity Prayer. See page **80** of the book.

Sessions Eleven, Twelve, and Thirteen

Goal: Seeing the whole sexual addiction picture.	**Material needed:** book and workbook, *Recovery From Sexual Addiction* books
Objective: Gain a deeper understanding of the host of conditions that contribute to or support sexual addiction.	**Chapters:** Six (book) Five (workbook)

From Chapter Six of the book and Chapter Five of the workbook:

Page #	**Action:** Read, do the exercises, and discuss.	
66-70 Book and **77-79** Workbook	**Primary Topic:** Role of Anger.	The purpose of this section is to understand that anger is a companion of the sexually-addicted man. Anger is a product of acting out, and, conversely, anger contributes to acting out. Often anger has, as does sexual addiction, its roots in childhood child/parent relationships.
	Discussion Topics:	**Discussion Points:**
70 Workbook	Childhood emotional nourishment.	Ask group members if they identify with any of the characterizations of fathers.
70-71 Workbook	Ely's Story.	Ask group members to comment on the type of love Ely's father had for Ely.
71-73 Workbook	Your family of origin.	Ask group members to: <ul><li>Complete the exercises and think about what it was like growing up in their families.</li><li>Share and discuss answers and insights to the questions.</li><li>Share feelings related to their relationship with their fathers.</li><li>Share the impact and feelings of not feeling valued.</li></ul>

73-76 Workbook	Childhood messages.	Ask group members to: • Complete the exercises and think about the messages they received from family members during childhood. • Share and discuss answers to the questions. • Share the feelings these messages generated. How did messages govern the assessment of one's self worth? • Share how deflating messages foster isolation and addiction. • What messages do group members send to their children?
66-67 Book **69** Workbook **77-79** Workbook	Role of Anger. Childhood abuse.	Ask group members to discuss the connection between anger and childhood family dysfunction and/or abuse. **Note:** Supplement by reading, "Sexual Iceberg," on page **69** of the workbook. **Note:** Supplement by completing the exercises under, "Role of Anger," on pages **77-79** of the workbook.
67-68 Book	Ralph's Story.	Ask group members: • What is the lesson presented in Ralph's Story? • Is his anger proportional to the importance of events? • What would it mean to realize one is not a bad person but a person who is struggling with a bad problem?
69 Book	Rules in the head. Sean's Story.	Ask group members: • If they have rules in their heads related to performance of others (wife, children, parents, work associates, etc.)? Give examples and discuss. • If others know they are being held accountable. • Do others have rules related to group member's performance? • What is the outcome of not being in control of one's environment?

| 69-70 Book | Anger at God. | Ask group members:
 • If they ever perceived themselves as being angry at God.
 • To characterize their anger at God—is it helpful or self-defeating?
 • Describe a reasonable expectation of God in one's life journey. |
| 70 Book | Anger alters mood. | Ask group members:
 • If they have experienced mood alteration during anger or rage.
 • How could anger substitute for acting out sexually? |

From Chapter Six of the book and Chapter Five of the workbook:

Page #	**Action:** Read, do the exercises, and discuss.	
70-73 Book	**Primary Topic:** Role of Anxiety.	The purpose of this section is to understand that anxiety is often a companion of the sexually-addicted man. Anxiety is both a product of and a contributor to acting-out behavior.
	Discussion Topics:	**Discussion Points:**
70 Book 80-81 Workbook	Sexual anxiety	Ask group members: • Does anxiety create sexual tension in their bodies? • What impact does anxiety have in fostering addiction? **Note:** Supplement by completing the exercises under, "The Role of Anxiety," on pages **80-81** of the workbook.
71 Book	Barry's Story.	Ask group members if they have difficulty facing normal activities until they masturbate to relieve anxiety.
71 Book	Situational anxiety.	Ask group members to describe situations that cause anxiety in their lives. Is acting out a solution to situational anxiety?

71-72 Book	Todd's Story.	Ask group members if they identify with Todd. How could Todd deal with his situational anxiety?
72 Book	Chronic anxiety.	Ask group members if living with anxiety has become a way of life.
72-73 Book	Mack's Story.	Ask group members if they identify with Mack.
73 Book	Treatment.	Ask group members to discuss the pros and cons of taking medication to control anxiety.

From Chapter Six of the book and Chapter Five of the workbook:

Page #	**Action:** Read, do the exercises, and discuss.	
73-79 Book	**Primary Topic:** Role of Depressed Mood.	The purpose of this section is to understand that depressed mood is often a companion of the sexually-addicted man. Depressed mood is both a product of and a contributor to acting-out behavior.
	Discussion Topics:	**Discussion Points:**
74-75 Book

82-83 Workbook | Chronic depressed mood. | Ask group members:
 • To read and discuss the "Role of Depressed Mood."
 • If they experience long periods of low-grade depressed mood?
 • What impact does depressed mood have in fostering addiction?

 Note: Supplement by reading and completing the exercises under, "The Role of Depressed Mood," on pages **82-83** of the workbook . |
| 76 Book | Addict's Life Scale | Ask group members:
 • To discuss the Addict's Life Scale concepts.
 • If they identify with the life scale values. |

85-86 Workbook	Your Life Scale	Ask group members: • To complete their life scales. • To discuss how the life scale relates to their lives. • To talk about their feelings associated with each level of their life scale. • How would they characterize their depressed mood. At what scale value do they live? • Is experiencing depressed mood destructive? • To discuss the consequences of living with depressed mood in their lives. • To discuss the pros and cons of taking medication to stabilize mood.
78 Book and **86-87** Workbook	Next steps.	Ask group members to: • Discuss the steps they can take to come out of their depressed mood. • How would the consistent application of the "40 activities" concept affect their marriage and sexual addiction. • How they could change their lives to live at "40." Record on large sheets of paper or on a board.
78-79 Book	Pete's Story.	Ask group members to share insights gained from Pete's Story. What decisions did Pete make to change his life?

From Chapter Six of the book and Chapter Five of the workbook:

Page #	**Action:** Read, do the exercises, and discuss.	
88-89 Workbook	**Primary Topic:** Role of Isolation.	The purpose of this section is to understand that isolation and loneliness are breeding grounds for depressed mood and sexual addiction.

	Discussion Topic:	Discussion Points:
88-90 Workbook	Isolation and loneliness.	Ask group members to: • Complete the exercises and think about what it is like to frequently experience isolation and loneliness. • Share answers and insights to the questions. • Share feelings related to isolation and loneliness. • Share the impact of isolation and loneliness in fostering addiction. • Share how men can come out of isolation. Record on large paper or a board.

From Chapter Six of the book and Chapter Five of the workbook:

Page #	**Action:** Read, do the exercises and discuss.	
92 Workbook	**Primary Topic:** Keep in Mind.	The purpose of this section is to review the tenets of this chapter.
	Discussion Topic.	**Discussion Points:**
92 Workbook	Share insights.	Ask group members to read and share insights.

Discuss key points group members learned from this chapter (end of the workbook Chapter Five). Insights gained become the fuel for changed behavior.

Handouts: None.

Homework Assignment: Read and complete Chapter Seven from the book and workbook.

End with the Serenity Prayer. See page **80** of the book.

GROUP PROGRAM
Sessions Fourteen and Fifteen

Goal: Reveal hope.	**Material needed:** book and workbook, *Recovery From Sexual Addiction* books
Objective: Gain deeper understanding of how the Lord loved other noted sinners. If He loved them, He can love the sexually-addicted man.	**Chapter:** Seven

From Chapter Seven of the book and workbook:

Page #	**Action:** Read, do exercises, and discuss.	
100-104 Workbook	**Primary Topic: Is There Hope?**	The purpose of this section is to understand that hope is available for the sexually-addicted man.
	Discussion Topics:	**Discussion Points:**
101 Workbook	Salvation history.	Ask group members if they are surprised to find biblical figures with an apparent sex addiction problem.
101-102 Workbook	King David.	Ask group members to ponder this: King David was a sinful man, but the Lord chose him to be at the head of Jesus' lineage. What does that imply for sexually-addicted men? **Note:** Ask group members to complete the exercises for each historical person presented as part of salvation history.
103 Workbook	Apostle Peter.	Ask group members to ponder this: Peter was a sinful man, but the Lord chose him to be the rock upon which He built His church. What does that imply for sexually-addicted men?

103-104 Workbook	Apostle Paul.	Ask group members: • To ponder this: Paul was a sinful man, but the Lord chose him to take the Word to the gentiles. What does that imply for sexually-addicted men? • Discuss the nature of the thorn in Paul's side. Could Paul's thorn have been addiction? If so, what does that imply for sexually-addicted men?
104 Workbook **84-85** Book	Change the dance.	Ask group members: • If they experience joy in their lives. Why? • If David, Peter, and Paul could change, can addicted men do the same? • Is God's grace sufficient for sexually-addicted men? **Note:** Supplement by reading and discussing, "Sonny's Story" and "Treatment Goals," on pages **84-85** of the book.

Discuss key points group members learned from this chapter (end of the workbook Chapter Seven) Insights gained become the fuel for changed behavior.

Handouts: None.

Homework Assignment: Read and complete Chapters Eight from the book and workbook.

End with the Serenity Prayer. See page **80** of the book.

GROUP PROGRAM
Sessions Sixteen and Seventeen

Goal: Awareness of choice.	**Material needed:** book and workbook, *Recovery From Sexual Addiction* books
Objective: Gain awareness of the possibility of changing the sexual-addiction dance.	**Chapter:** Eight

From Chapter Eight of the book and workbook:

Page #	**Action:** Read, do the exercises, and discuss.	
89 Book	**Primary Topic:** Change the Dance	The purpose of this section is to understand that what has been learned to date serves as a platform to change the sexual addiction dance.
	Discussion Topic:	**Discussion Points**
89 Book	Awareness leads to choices.	Ask group members to: • Discuss "awareness leads to choices." Do group members agree or disagree? • Ponder this question: While I did not ask to become sexually addicted, is it time to make an adult decision to change my sexual-addiction dance?
107-113 Workbook	Summary Review. Affect on my life. The origin of my addiction. Factors that keep me addicted. Role of anger. Role of anxiety. Role of low-grade depression. Role of isolation. Exceptions.	Ask group members to: • Complete the exercises and think about the totality of what keeps each man sexually addicted. • Share and discuss any new insight gained or additional information discovered since recording one's sexual inventory in Chapter One. • Share feelings after completing each exercise. • Share insights gained from reviewing the full sexual-addiction picture. • Answer the question, "Am I ready to move on?"

From Chapter Eight of the book and workbook:

Page #	**Action:** Read, do the exercises, and discuss.	
89-95 Book	**Primary Topic:** Changing the Dance—New Steps.	The purpose of this section is to identify essential new steps needed to change the sexual addiction dance.
	Discussion Topics:	**Discussion Points:**
89-93 Book	Changing the Dance— New Steps. Commitment. Awareness as part of commitment. Bill's Story.	Ask group members to: • Read and think about what changing the sexual-addiction dance means. • Discuss the difference between "white-knuckling" and a "high-level commitment." • Describe "white-knuckling" efforts that are not working. • Describe what a "high-level commitment" would look like. • Discuss what an "irrevocable decision" means to the sexually-addicted man. • Discuss the handout, Stash. • Discuss the meaning of "stash." • Share if they are willing to take a recovery step by trashing all stash. • Share insights gained from this section.
115 Workbook		**Note:** Supplement by completing the exercises, "Changing the Dance" on pages **115** of the workbook.

93-94 Book	Recognize that addiction causes more pain than pleasure.	Ask group members to: • Read and compare long-term pain of guilt and shame to the short-term pleasure of acting out. • Discuss the difference between long-term pain and a short-term pleasure. • Answer the question: Is my equation out of balance? • Answer the question: If my pain is greater than my pleasure, why would I want to continue to accept that pain? • Share insights gained from this section. **Note:** Supplement by completing the exercise, "Recognize that addiction causes more pain than pleasure," on pages **116-117** of the workbook.
116-117 Workbook		
94-95 Book	Address Environmental Temptation. Jim's Story. Jay's Story. Matt's Story.	Ask group members to: • Read and think about how environmental temptations keep men trapped in sexual addiction. • Discuss what environmental factors need to be addressed when a high-level commitment is made to end sexually addictive thinking, fantasy, and behavior. • Discuss each story as it relates to addressing environmental temptation. **Note:** Supplement by completing the exercises, "Address Environmental Temptation" on page **117** of the workbook.
117 Workbook		

Discuss key points group members learned from this chapter (end of the workbook Chapter Eight). Insights gained become the fuel for changed behavior.

Handouts: Stash.

Homework Assignment: Read and complete Chapters Nine from the book and workbook.

End with the Serenity Prayer. See page **80** of the book.

Sessions Eighteen and Nineteen

Goal: Choosing a healthy life style.	Material needed: book and workbook, *Recovery From Sexual Addiction* books
Objective: Understand choices that constitute a healthy life style free of sex addiction.	Chapter: Nine

From Chapter Seven of the book:

Page #	Action: Read and discuss.	
97-116 Book	Topic: What is a Healthy Life Style?	The purpose of this section is to define four elements of a healthy life style.
	Discussion Topic:	**Discussion Points:**
97 Book	Why is changing one's life style important?	Ask group members to project how a healthier life style would: • Impact sexually-addictive behavior. • Raise depressed mood • Enable a new relationship with God. • Enable feelings of peace and joy. • Reduce feelings of shame. Ask group members: • Why a healthy life style is essential to sexual addiction recovery? • What would a healthy life style look like? • How would a healthy life style complement a high-level commitment to end sexual thinking, fantasy, and behavior? • What are the benefits of living a healthy life style?

From Chapter Nine of the book and workbook:

Page #	**Action:** Read, do the exercises, and discuss.	
97-101 Book	**Primary Topic:** Coming Out of Isolation.	The purpose of this section is to explore the steps that define coming out of isolation.
	Discussion Topic:	**Discussion Points:**
98-99 Book **120-121** Workbook	Coming out of isolation by cultivating a strong male friendship.	Ask group members: • Why does coming out of isolation include cultivating a strong male friendship? • To discuss whether cultivating a strong male friendship is easy or difficult. Why? • Share insights gained from this section. **Note:** Supplement by completing the exercises under, "Coming Out of Isolation," and "Coming out of isolation by cultivating a strong male friendship," on pages **120-121** of the workbook.
98 Book **121-123** Workbook	Coming out of isolation by improving family relationships.	Ask group members why coming out of isolation includes improving family relationships. **Note:** Supplement by completing the exercises under, "Coming out of isolation by improving family relationships," on pages **121-123** of the workbook.
99 Book **123-124** Workbook	Coming out of isolation by improving relationships with spouse and children.	Ask group members why coming out of isolation includes improving relationships with one's spouse and children. **Note:** Supplement by completing the exercises under, "Coming out of isolation by improving relationships with spouse and children," on pages **123-124** of the workbook.

99-101 Book	I know that I have intimacy in my marriage when…	Ask group members: • Why is fostering non-sexual intimacy essential to improving relationships? • What the difference is in relationship building between non-sexual intimacy and sexual intimacy?
101 Book	Compartmentalization	Ask group members: • Do they identify with the concept of compartmentalization? • Do women have it right?
101-103 Book	Disclosure	Ask group members: • Have they disclosed their sexual addiction to their partner? • Is there more to be disclosed? • How much disclosure is appropriate?

From Chapter Nine of the book and workbook:

Page #	**Action:** Read, do the exercises, and discuss.	
103-104 Book	**Primary Topic:** Giving-up Depressed Mood	The purpose of this section is to explore how giving-up depressed mood supports sexual addiction recovery.
	Discussion Topic:	**Discussion Points:**
103-104 Book	Choose to take steps to live at "great to be alive," (forty-point benchmark mood level).	Ask group members: • Why giving up a depressed mood is essential to sexual addiction recovery? • What would living life closer to "**40**" look like? • Answer the question: What activities would I incorporate into my life to live closer to "**40**?" • How would giving up a depressed mood complement a high-level commitment to end sexual thinking, fantasy, and behavior? • What are the consequences of giving up a depressed mood?
125-127 Workbook		**Note:** Supplement by completing the exercises under, "Giving-up depressed mood," and "Choose to take steps to live at '**40**,'" on pages **125-127** of the workbook.

From Chapter Nine of the book and workbook:

Page #	Action: Read, do the exercises, and discuss.	
104 Book	**Primary Topic:** Develop a Support Network	The purpose of this section is to explore how an effective support network is an essential step in overcoming sexual addiction.
	Discussion Topic:	**Discussion Points:**
104 Book **130** Workbook	Twelve-step program and accountability.	Ask group members: • Why it is essential to develop a network to support sexual addiction recovery? • How would a support network complement a high-level commitment to end sexual thinking, fantasy, and behavior? • What would a support network look like? • If they attend one or more sex addiction Twelve-Step Programs. • How frequently do they attend Twelve-Step programs? • Do they have an accountability partner? Describe the relationship. **Note:** Supplement by completing the exercises under, "Develop a Support Network" on page **130** of the workbook

From Chapter Nine of the book:

Page #	Action: Read and discuss.	
105-108 Book	**Primary Topic:** Interventions.	The purpose of this section is to provide interventions that men have found useful in times of temptation.

	Discussion Topics:	Discussion Points:
105-108 Book	Interventions and planning ahead.	Ask group members to: • Choose interventions that would support their recovery and explain why. • Discuss why the application of interventions differs before and after making a high-level commitment. • Prepare two cards and share the contents of these cards.

From Chapter Nine of the book:

Page #	**Action:** Read and discuss.	
109-110 Book	**Primary Topic:** New Behaviors in Place of Old Behaviors.	The purpose of this section is to suggest that, on the road to recovery, it is easier and more effective if new behaviors are adopted, rather than "white-knuckle" the removal of old behaviors.
	Discussion Topics:	Discussion Points:
109 Book	New Behaviors in Place of Old Behaviors.	Ask group members: • Why it is more prudent to introduce new behaviors in one's life in contrast to backing off old behaviors? • What new behaviors support sexual addiction recovery for each man? • What insights were gained from this section?
109 Book	Jude's Story. George's Story.	What new behaviors did Jude and George introduce to change their sexual addiction dance?
109 Book	Backing off behaviors.	Ask group members: • What behaviors would they find easier to give up? • What behaviors would they find difficult to give up?

110 Book	Glen's Story.	Ask group members: • What behaviors did Glen find easier to give up? • How does adopting new behaviors help the sexually-addicted man?

From Chapter Nine of the book:

Page #	**Action:** Read and discuss.	
111-115 Book	**Primary Topic:** Spirituality.	The purpose of this section is to explore why recovery is deepened through a relationship with God.
	Discussion Topics:	**Discussion Points:**
111-113 Book	Spirituality and Dave's Story.	Ask group members: • Is a healthy relationship with God essential to sexual addiction recovery? • What would a healthy relationship with God look like? • How would a healthy relationship with God foster a high-level commitment to end sexual thinking, fantasy, and behavior? • What are the consequences of a close relationship with God? • What insights were gained from Dave's Story?
113 Book	What does my addiction have to do with God?	Ask group members: • What would it mean to depend on God to satisfy one's greatest need rather than depending on sex as one's greatest need? • How would a positive relationship with God help the addict to come out of isolation?

113-114 Book	Jason's Story.	Ask group members: • To discuss the transitions Jason made to change his addiction dance and his relationship with God. • Why did nothing work for Jason until he made the decision to turn to God? • What insights were gained from Jason's Story?
114-115 Book	Committed and genuine relationship with God.	Ask group members: • What is a committed relationship with God? • How is a committed relationship with God different than just going to church each Sunday? • Why is a committed relationship with God like finding the Holy Grail?

From Chapter Nine of the book:

Page #	**Action:** Read and discuss.	
115 Book	**Primary Topic:** Surrender.	The purpose of this section is to understand that surrendering to the will of God gives power to the sexually-addicted man.
	Discussion Topic:	**Discussion Points:**
115 Book	Surrender one's will to God.	Ask group members: • Why does surrendering to the will of God give power to the sexually-addicted man? • How does surrendering freedom result in becoming truly free? • What insights were gained from this section?

Discuss key points group members learned from this chapter (end of the workbook Chapter Nine). Insights gained become the fuel for changed behavior.

Handouts: Distribute the exercise, *Prepared to Live a Changed Life* exercise, Appendix B to group members.

Homework Assignment: Read and complete, *Prepared to Live a Changed Life* exercise. Ask the group to be prepared to discuss their answers in the next session.

End with the Serenity Prayer. See page **80** of the book.

Goal: Commitment to change.	**Material needed:** *Preparing to Live a Changed Life* document, Appendix B.
Objective: Understand what a continuing commitment to end sexual addiction looks like.	**Chapter:** The rest of your life.

Preparing to Live a Changed Life

Ask group members to:

- Share answers from the "change" part of the exercise (Appendix B).
- Discuss why they chose their answers.
- Select three leading changes they plan to address. Limit the focus at this time. If group members can remain committed to three changes, progress will be significant. Some important change items are: come out of isolation, live a healthy lifestyle, maintain a high-level commitment, and deepen one's relationship with God. Group members may wish to address one or more of these in different ways.
- Discuss insights gained from this exercise.

Ask group members to:

- Address the question: "On my recovery journey, I have to give up _____"
- Share answers and why each chose their answers.
- Discuss fears of giving up sexual thinking, fantasies, and behaviors that they have lived with for so many years.
- Share how they will keep themselves accountable to live a changed life.

Discuss next steps:

This program is only the beginning of the recovery journey. For most men, the journey will take several years and perhaps even the rest of one's life. It is essential for each group member to have a continuing support program.

Ask group members to discuss:

- Attending Sex Addicts Anonymous or another Twelve-Step program
  (See Appendix A: Counseling and Support Programs in the book).
- Reading (See Appendix A: Counseling and Support Programs in the book).
- Maintaining an accountability partner.
- Continuing individual or group therapy.
- Initiating marital therapy.

- Enabling spirituality in one's life.
- Attending specialized treatment programs.

Homework Assignment: Continue to attend Twelve-Step programs, meet frequently with one's accountability partner, and continue a counseling relationship as needed.

End with the Serenity Prayer. See page **80** of the book.

Appendix A: Trash Stash

There are many changes you may choose to make as you journey toward recovery, and they will come in due time. There is, however, a significant step you can take today that will serve to make a statement of commitment and be a positive step to reduce your acting-out behavior.

The first step is to "trash stash." Sexually-addicted men frequently pledge to stop their acting-out behavior. However, most do not get rid of all the crutches that facilitate acting out. Stash is the hidden pornographic magazine and videos; sex toys; articles of clothing; the computer URLs that leads to pornography, or the telephone number which the addicted man keeps in case of temptation or sexual urge to act out.

Trashing stash is a firm commitment to remove all lust traps in one's possession. It doesn't mean getting rid of some or most on one's stash, it means getting rid of *all* of it. A commitment to remove stash is not easily made. It means parting with the "keys to the addiction car." Parting with stash is not recovery but an early step toward recovery.

Your commitment to trash your stash includes a plan to remove or destroy stash.

Complete the exercise:

My Stash is:

1.

_____
_____
_____
_____

2.

_____
_____
_____
_____

My commitment plan is:

1.

_____

_____

_____

_____

2.

_____

_____

_____

_____

Appendix B: Preparing to Live a Changed Life

Choosing a journey free of sex addiction involves changes in how you think, feel, and behave. Although healing ultimately brings a better life, it also threatens to permanently alter life as you have known it. Your relationships, your position in the world, even your sense of identity may change. Old coping patterns may no longer work. When you make the commitment to heal, you risk losing much of what is familiar. As a result, one part of you may want to heal while another resists change.

To prepare to accept change, it is a good idea to cognitively acknowledge where change is likely to take place. Take a few minutes to think about parts of your life that may change as you heal. Then fill out the following change inventory. Start with the areas that are most important to you.

If I sincerely continue to my commitment to healing, the following will probably change:

How my feelings may change (entitlement, shame, guilt, anger, anxiety, depressed mood, attitudes, beliefs, self-image):

1. _____

2. _____

3. _____

4. _____

5. _____

6. _____

How I will change behaviors related to isolation (addiction cycle/addiction ritual/fantasies):

1. _____

2. _____

3. _____

4. _____

How my lifestyle will change (habits, patterns, leisure-time activities, types of friends, efforts to live more often at "**40**"):

1. _____

2. _____

3. _____

4. _____

5. _____

6. _____

How my relationship with my partner will change:

1. _____

2. _____

3. _____

4. _____

How my relationships with my children, siblings, parents, friends will change:

1. _____

2. _____

3. _____

4. _____

How my continuing recovery program will change (Twelve-Step program, counseling, accountability partner, strong male friend):

1. _____

2. _____

3. _____

4. _____

How my spirituality will change:

1. _____

2. _____

3. _____

4. _____

How areas of my life might change:

1. _____

2. _____

3. _____

4. _____

Look over the lists you have made. Put a check mark next to three items where change is likely to occur first. Your commitment should start with these items. As you grow, return to your inventory and add other items that you wish to address in your life.

Also, identify some of your potential losses. Without too much thinking, fill in the following sentences—as many times as you can: (Example: On my recovery journey, I have to give up:

- People feeling sorry for me
- Blaming my parents for my problems
- Feeling that I am not worthy of God's love, etc.

Of the things you would have to give up—include such items as fantasies, "stash" (hidden porn magazines, reserved URL's), isolation behaviors, etc.

On my recovery journey, I have to give up

_____

_____

_____

_____

On my recovery journey, I have to give up

_____

_____

_____

_____

On my recovery journey, I have to give up

_____

_____

_____

_____

On my recovery journey, I have to give up

_____

_____

_____

_____

On my recovery journey, I have to give up

_____

_____

_____

_____

On my recovery journey, I have to give up

_____

_____

_____

_____